BABY-LED WEANING RECIPES BOOK

Best Nourishing Recipes for Every Stage of Starting Solids for your Baby while Catering for the Whole Family too.

Angelina Marsh

© Copyright 2021 Angelina Marsh

All rights reserved. The content contained within this book may not be reproduced, duplicated or transmitted without direct written permission from the author or the publisher.

Under no circumstances will any blame or legal responsibility be held against the publisher, or author, for any damages, reparation, or monetary loss due to the information contained within this book. Either directly or indirectly.

Disclaimer Notice

Please note the information contained within this document is for educational and entertainment purposes only. All effort has been executed to present accurate, up to date, and reliable, complete information. No warranties of any kind are declared or implied. Readers acknowledge that the author is not engaging in the rendering of legal, financial, medical or professional advice.

Please consult a licensed professional before attempting any techniques outlined in this book.

By reading this document, the reader agrees that under no circumstances is the author responsible for any losses, direct or indirect, which are incurred as a result of the use of information contained within this document, including, but not limited to errors, omissions, or inaccuracies.

Table of Contents

Introduction 1

Sweet Potato Baby Food: BLW-Style and Pureed............. 2

Easy Avocado Puree 5

Banana Puree Baby Food 7

Easiest Butternut Squash Puree 9

Instant Pot Applesauce 12

Bean Dip Recipe... 15

Rice Cakes 16

Andrew's Carrot Muffins 17

Home-made Oatcakes 19

Lamb and Spinach Lasagne – SFF 20

Cinnamon-Banana Pancakes 22

Veggie Parmesan Bread... 24

Overnight Blueberry Oats... 26

Freezer-Friendly Spinach Waffles 27

Grinch Mini Muffins for Baby + Toddler 30

Broccoli Egg Cups 35

Avocado Toast with Hard Boiled Egg 37

Almond Butter + Banana with Hemp Seed Sprinkles 39

Wholesome Blueberry Sheet Pan Pancakes 41

Easy Cheesy Egg Roll-Ups 44

Whole Grain Pumpkin Waffle Dippers 46

Golden Milk Waffles for Baby + Toddlers + Kids 49

Easy Blender Spinach Pancakes for Baby + Toddler (Allergy Friendly!) 52

Blender Muffin Recipes 55

Spiced Blender Pancakes 60

4 Baked Oatmeal Cups for Baby, Toddler + Kids 63

Sweet Potato Waffles for Baby and Toddler 67

Avocado + Blueberry Yummy Toddler Mini Muffins 70

Spiced Blender Pancakes 72

Lunch Recipes 75

Cheesy Broccoli Quinoa Bites 75

Mini Bagel Pizzas with Pepper "Sprinkles" 77

Tortellini On-a-Stick with Marinara Dipping Sauce 79

Curry Pasta Salad for Baby + Toddler 81

Summer Pesto Finger Salad for Baby + Toddler 85

Green Finger Salad for Baby + Toddler 87

Snacks Recipes.. 89

Veggie-Loaded Hummus for Baby and Toddler 89

Warm Peach Chunks with Nutmeg for Baby & Toddler . 93

Healthy Strawberry Cream Cheese Dip........................... 95

Easy Whole Grain Baked Cheese Crackers 97

Dinner Recipes..100

Crispy Herb Salmon Bites for Baby + Toddler 100

Easy Veggie "Fried" Rice for Baby + Toddler 103

Taco Tuesday for Baby..105

Mexican Sweet Potato Boats..108

Baked Seasoned Chicken Tenders..................................111

Baked Seasoned Tofu Finger Food Nuggets..................114

Kale Pesto Chicken Quesadilla 117

Baby's First Bolognese.. 119

Easy-Peasy 5 Veggie Pasta for Baby................................ 121

Chunky Summer Veggie Pasta... 124

Crispy White Fish with Pineapple & Avocado Chunks .. 128

Family-Favorite Pumpkin Pasta 131

Kid-Friendly Pumpkin Risotto 134

Butternut Squash Mac N Cheese 137

Healthy Chicken Nuggets with Green Bean "Fries" 140

Spinach Waffles.. 144

Introduction

So glad you were able to get this recipe book.

These baby-led weaning recipes are nutritious first finger foods for babies from 6 months of age.

Low in salt and soft in texture you will find easy BLW meal ideas, baby snacks & breakfasts

Introducing solids should be fun, not stressful, I hope your little one enjoys these baby led weaning ideas.

All my BLW recipes are below, but also don't forget to check out my essential guide titled "Guide to Baby-Led Weaning: Most Useful Guide to Integrating Solid Foods, Raising Happy, Independent Eaters and Helping Your Baby Grow with Confidence" as your baby may be able to join in the family meal.

Most popular BLW recipes in this book includes Sweet Potato Baby Food: Blw-Style And Pureed, Sweet Potato Waffles for Baby and Toddler, Mini Bagel Pizzas with Pepper "Sprinkles" and many more.

RECIPES

Sweet Potato Baby Food: BLW-Style and Pureed

Prep Time: 5 minutes | Cook Time: 22 minutes

Total Time: 27 minutes | Yield: 2-4 servings

Category: Side | Method: Roasting

Cuisine: American

You can serve this as wedges, a thick mash, or a thinner puree to your baby or toddler. (Adults will love the wedges too!)

Ingredients

- 1 large orange-fleshed sweet potato (or garnet yam)
- 1 tablespoon olive oil

Instructions

1. Preheat oven to 400 degrees and line a rimmed baking sheet with foil. Coat with nonstick spray.
2. Wash and dry the sweet potato.

3. Cut in half, then cut lengthwise into strips. Cut each strip in half again until each is about 1/2-inch thick. Slice in half horizontally if the sweet potato is very long. (Each strip should be about the size of your finger.)
4. Place into a bowl and toss with the olive oil.
5. Spread onto prepared baking sheet and roast for 22-25 minutes or until soft.
6. Let cool slightly and serve as is for a BLW-style finger food.
7. To serve as a thick mash, remove skin and mash with a fork one at a time or in a larger portion in a food processor or blender.
8. To serve as a thinner sweet potato puree, mash with a fork and add 1 tablespoon warm water at a time to reach the desired consistency.

Notes

- Store any leftovers in an airtight container for 3-5 days in the fridge.
- You can sprinkle with salt for babies over 1 and any adults.
- Add crushed dried rosemary OR cinnamon for additional flavor.
- Spread the wedges out on the baking sheet so they aren't overlapping. This will ensure even cooking.
- Poke a wedge with a fork or small knife at the lower end of the baking time to see if it's very soft.

Easy Avocado Puree

Prep Time: 5 minutes | Total Time: 5 minutes

Yield: 1 cup (serving is 1 tbsp) | Category: Baby food

Method: Blender | Cuisine: American

This easy baby food is rich in healthy fats, super smooth, and has a mellow flavor. This is a great puree to make when you're eating something like tacos...so you can have some too!

Ingredients

- ripe avocado

Instructions

1. Cut the avocado in half and scoop out the flesh. You'll need at least 1 cup to do this in a blender.
2. Add to a blender. Start on low and blend smooth, adding a little water, breastmilk, or formula as needed to thin and create a smooth consistency.
3. Serve immediately.
4. To store, place puree into small food storage containers and squeeze fresh lemon juice over top.

You'll want any exposed part of the puree to be in contact with some lemon juice to prevent browning.

Notes

- To do this with a fork, place as much or as little avocado onto a plate. Mash with a fork to reach the desired consistency, thinning with water, breastmilk or formula as desired.
- To freeze, stir 1 tablespoon fresh lemon juice into the mash and spoon into an ice cube tray. Freeze. Transfer frozen cubes into a freezer storage bag for up to 3 months. Thaw overnight in the fridge in an airtight container. (You can also freeze directly in a freezer bag.)
- Leave as a thicker mash for older babies.
- Spread onto toast sticks (about the size of your finger) for BLW-style feeding or offer a preloaded spoon.
- Mix with banana puree, sweet potato puree, pureed beans, or any other food you like.

Banana Puree Baby Food

Prep Time: 5 minutes | Total Time: 5 minutes

Yield: Makes about 1 cup (serving is 1 tbsp)

Category: Baby Food | Method: Blender

Cuisine: American

Use a ripe banana with at least some brown spots for the best flavor in this puree.

Ingredients

- 1 ripe banana (about 1 cup sliced)

Instructions

1. Slice banana to measure out about 1 cup.
2. Add to a blender. Blend until very smooth, stopping to scrape down the sides as needed.
3. Serve immediately.

Notes

- To store, place into small airtight storage containers and store in the fridge.
- To freeze, place into an ice cube tray, freeze, then transfer frozen cubes to a freezer bag and freeze for up to 3 months. Thaw overnight in an airtight container in the fridge.
- To make a thicker banana puree, you can simply mash a ripe banana until mostly smooth using a fork or potato masher.
- Add a sprinkle of cinnamon for additional flavor.
- To help prevent the puree from browning, you can add a few drops of an acid such as fresh lemon or orange juice.
- Mix with whole milk plain yogurt, baby oatmeal, mashed avocado, sweet potato, or any other baby food you like as desired.

Easiest Butternut Squash Puree

Prep Time: 10 minutes | Cook Time: 18 minutes

Total Time: 28 minutes | Yield: Makes about 2 cups puree

Category: Baby Food | Method: Roasting

Cuisine: American

You can make this puree to feed to a baby or toddler, or as a simple side dish for the whole family to share.

Ingredients

- 1 medium butternut squash
- 1 tablespoon olive oil

Instructions

1. Preheat oven to 375 degrees F. Remove the peel of the squash with a vegetable peeler or with a knife.
2. Cut the "neck", or the skinnier part of the squash into 1/2-inch rounds and dice.
3. Place on a greased foil-lined baking sheet in one even layer and bake for 18-22 minutes or until soft when poked a fork.

4. Add to a blender and puree, adding 1/4-1/2 cup water as needed to make a smooth puree.
5. Serve or store in an airtight container/s in the fridge for 3-5 days. Or portion into an ice cube tray and freeze, then transfer frozen cubes to a zip top storage bag and freeze for up to 3 months.

Notes

- Roast the squash until soft when poked with a fork.
- Add water slowly to reach the desired smooth consistency.
- Stop and scrape down the sides of the blender as needed.
- Stir in 1/2 teaspoon cinnamon, 1/4 teaspoon ground ginger, 1/8 teaspoon Chinese Five Spice, 1/2 teaspoon cumin, or 1/2 teaspoon Pumpkin Pie Spice if desired to add more flavor.
- Stir in apple butter or applesauce to make a slightly sweeter apple-butternut squash puree. (This is a nice topping for pancakes and waffles!)

- You can serve it as is, or you can use it in Butternut Squash Muffins, in Baby Oatmeal with Butternut Squash, you can stir it into plain yogurt, spread it on toast, stir it into Marinara Sauce, or use it in quesadillas.

Instant Pot Applesauce

Prep Time: 10 minutes | Cook Time: 8 minutes

Total Time: 18 minutes | Yield: About 1 quart

Category: Snack | Method: Instant Pot

Cuisine: American

You can peel or not peel the apples, depending on your preference.

Ingredients

- 6–7 medium apples (about 8 cups chopped)
- 1/2 cup water
- 1 teaspoon cinnamon, optional

Instructions

1. Chop the apples so they're about 1/2-1 inch in size. It's okay if they aren't 100% uniform in size.
2. Add to the instant pot. Add water. Seal.
3. Set to cook for 8 minutes on high.

4. When the cooking is done, either do a quick manual release OR let the pressure naturally release. Both are fine.
5. Mash or puree as desired. To get the skins smooth and well-blended, I prefer to add the cooked apples to a blender and blend smooth. You can use a potato masher to make chunky applesauce or puree in a food processor.
6. Stir in cinnamon, if desired.

Notes

- Once cooled, store in an airtight container in the fridge for a week or in a freezer-safe container in the freezer for up to 3 months. Let thaw in the fridge and stir before serving.
- Use firm cooking apples such as Jonathan, Cortland, Granny Smith, Pink Lady, or Jonagold.
- To make a chunkier applesauce, peel the apples before cooking and mash lightly with a potato masher.

- Add cinnamon or fresh lemon juice to taste after the applesauce is cooked and blended.
- You can blend this in a blender, food processor, or with an immersion blender.
- Store finished applesauce in airtight containers in the fridge for up to a week, or in the freezer for up to 3 months

Bean Dip Recipe

We let them sneak on occasionally just to make the place look purty.

A 'dip' recipe but makes a nice thick and clingy spread, so, it can be put on rice cakes, toast or used as sandwich filling.

Ingredients

- 1 tin of pinto beans
- 2 tbsp lime juice
- 1 tomato [skinned and seeded]
- 1 minced garlic clove
- bit of ground cumin
- handful [or less] parsley
- spring onion
- seasoning optional!
- whizz all up in a blender or food processor

Rice Cakes

Ingredients

- 150g/5¼oz cooked Thai fragrant rice
- 1 free-range egg, beaten
- 2 spring onions, finely chopped
- ½ red pepper, finely chopped
- drizzle soy sauce
- 1-2 tbsp olive oil

Instructions

1. Preheat the oven to 220C/425F/Gas 7.
2. Place the cooked rice into a large bowl. Stir in the beaten egg along with the spring onions, pepper and soy sauce.
3. Heat the oil in a small to medium non-stick frying pan. Spoon the rice mixture into the pan and press down. Fry for about two minutes. Transfer the pan to the oven and cook for a further 10-12 minutes.
4. Remove from the oven and allow to cool slightly. Turn the cake out and cut into wedges to serve.

Andrew's Carrot Muffins

Probably noooot really called Andrew, in fact, but this email wasn't signed so Andrew is the only nominative detail I can glean from our correspondence. For the record, I think that if you want to make your own buttermilk you just mix equal amounts of natural yoghurt and semi-skimmed milk. I think...

Says 'Andrew':

"I reckon you could swop carrot for courgette, pepper, onion, etc, though probably fry them a bit first.

Also, use any different cheese and herbs, and I'm sure normal milk would work, if you can't get buttermilk.

Ingredients

- 1 carrot, grated
- 15 stalks parsley, chopped
- 60g cheddar, grated
- 220g self-raising flour
- 1 egg
- 3/4 cup buttermilk (about 150ml, I think?)
- 1/2 cup vegetable oil

Instructions

1. Preheat oven to 180c.
2. Mix carrot, parsley, cheese and flour.
3. In another bowl, whisk egg, buttermilk and oil.
4. Add this to dry ingredients and mix.
5. Spoon into muffin cases (makes 12) and bake for 20-25 mins."

Home-made Oatcakes

Ingredients

- 8oz oatmeal
- 1/4 teaspoon baking powder
- 1 dessertspoonful of melted fat,
- hot water
- a good pinch of salt.

Instructions

Mix all the dry ingredients together with a well in the middle and pour in the fat. Blend in enough hot water to make a stiff paste then knead and roll out as thinly as possible. Cut into triangles and bake on a floured tin at 200 degrees until the ends curl up and the cakes are crisp. Alternatively, bake them on a hot girdle or frying pan.

Lamb and Spinach Lasagne – SFF

Ingredients

- 2 x 400g packs of lamb mince
- 2 bags of baby leaf spinach
- 2 tins chopped tomatoes
- 3 peppers
- 2 onions
- lasagne pasta sheets
- some grated cheddar
- cheese sauce packet
- a few chives
- squidge of tomato puree

Instructions

1. Chop and gently fry the peppers and onions. Remove from the pan, (a VERY big pan), and then brown the mince. Replace the peppers and onions and a bag of the spinache, both tins of tomatoes and the squidge of puree. I usually add a bit of cayenne pepper or chilli powder too at this point.

2. Let it all simmer and make up your cheese sauce and grate the cheddar.
3. Grease a huge lasagne type baking thing (I have a big oval glass one that lets me see my layers).
4. Place pasta sheets followed by mince mixture then the raw spinach. Follow for two or three layers.
5. Pour the cheese sauce on top followed by the grated cheddar, a few spinach leaves for decoration and some chives.
6. Place in the oven for a few hours on about 180. (or when it looks done, just test with a fork).
7. I always make one this big so that I can freeze portions for dd2 as it's her favourite.

Cinnamon-Banana Pancakes

These sweet cakes contain no added sugar and no flour. Serve plain or spread with a thin layer of peanut butter or almond butter for an even more substantial snack or breakfast. Refrigerate these pancakes for up to 3 days. Reheat briefly, or just serve cold or at room temperature.

Ingredients

- 1 egg
- 1 ripe banana, mashed (about ½ cup)
- 1/8 tsp. ground cinnamon
- 1 Tbs. unsalted butter.

Instructions

1. Break the egg into a medium bowl and beat with a fork. Add the mashed banana and cinnamon, and stir to combine. The batter will seem very runny.
2. Melt the butter on a large griddle or in a large, preferably nonstick, skillet. Drop the banana batter by tablespoonfuls onto the pan and cook until golden brown and cooked through, about 3

minutes on the first side and 1 to 2 minutes on the second. Cool and serve.

Veggie Parmesan Bread

Tote this savory snack to daycare or on the road. It also makes a satisfying breakfast. If you're making this bread for toddlers, big kids, and/or grown-ups (and you should!) add 1 teaspoon of salt to the batter.

Ingredients

- Nonstick cooking spray
- 1 cup all-purpose flour
- ½ cup cornmeal
- ½ cup grated Parmesan cheese
- 1 tablespoon baking powder
- ½ teaspoon baking soda
- 3 eggs
- 1 cup buttermilk
- 1/3 cup canola or olive oil
- 1 cup grated zucchini
- 1 cup chopped cooked spinach (start with frozen, defrost, and drain well)
- ½ cup grated carrots

Instructions

1. Preheat the oven to 350°F. Spray a 9 x 5-inch loaf pan with cooking spray.
2. In a large bowl, whisk together the flour, cornmeal, Parmesan, baking powder, and baking soda.
3. In a small bowl, whisk together the eggs, buttermilk, and canola oil.
4. Add the wet ingredients to the dry ingredients, and stir to combine. Stir in the zucchini, spinach, and carrots. Transfer to the prepared loaf pan.
5. Bake the bread for 45 minutes, or until a toothpick inserted into the center of the loaf comes out clean. Cool on a wire rack for 15 minutes. Remove the bread from the pan and cool completely on the rack. To serve, slice and cube. Store in the fridge.

Overnight Blueberry Oats

This recipe for easy overnight oats flavored with colorful blueberries and is perfect for baby 6 months and up.

Ingredients

- 1/4 cup blueberries, frozen
- 1/2 cup milk of choice – regular, almond, oat, etc
- 1/4 tsp cinnamon
- 1/3 cup old-fashioned oats
- 1/4 tsp chia seeds, optional

Instructions

1. In a blender, add in the blueberries, milk and cinnamon and blend until smooth.
2. In a small bowl or jar, add in the oats and chia seeds and pour in the blueberry milk. Stir and cover with a lid or saran wrap. Place in the fridge and let sit overnight.
3. Take out the oats, stir and serve. I like to serve them chunky, so baby can have more to grab onto.

Freezer-Friendly Spinach Waffles

Warm and wholesome waffles made with nutrient packed spinach!

Course: Breakfast | Cuisine: American

Prep Time: 5 Minutes | Cook Time: 15 Minutes

Servings: 16 Small Waffles | Calories: 94kcal

Ingredients

- 2 cups white whole wheat flour (see flour notes)
- 1 tbsp baking powder
- 1 tsp cinnamon
- 1/4 tsp salt
- 2 large eggs
- 1 cup milk
- 1/4 cup olive oil or melted coconut oil
- 1/4 cup applesauce
- 1/2 tsp vanilla extract
- 1 cup packed spinach

Instructions

1. Preheat waffle iron to medium heat.
2. In a medium bowl, stir together the flour, baking powder, cinnamon and salt.
3. In a blender, add in the eggs, milk, oil, applesauce, vanilla extract and spinach. Blend for 1 minute on medium speed or until the spinach is completely blended.
4. Add the spinach mixture to the flour mixture and stir until just combined.
5. Pour waffle mixture onto waffle iron in 1/4 cup increments and bake according to waffle makers instructions.
6. Serve or store in an air-tight container in the fridge or freezer.

Notes

Freezer-Friendly: take any leftovers and place in a freezer zip-lock baggie and freeze. To reheat, place in toaster and toast until warm. Will last 2-3 months in the freezer.

Notes on Flour: you can use all-purpose, white whole wheat or whole wheat flour in any combination that you prefer, I will usually use a combo of 1 cup all-purpose and 1 cup whole wheat or 2 cups white wheat flour. You can also make these gluten-free using a gluten-free flour mix (this is our favorite). If using whole wheat flour, you may need to add in extra milk to thin it out as whole wheat flour is extra absorbent.

Notes on Milk: if your dough is too thick, add in up to 1 more cup of milk. Depending on which flour you use, you may need more milk.

Grinch Mini Muffins for Baby + Toddler

Made with no added sugar and packed with spinach – these muffins can be served for breakfast, lunch, snack or even an age-appropriate dessert!

Course: Breakfast | Cuisine: American

Prep Time: 10 Minutes | Cook Time: 15 Minutes

Total Time: 25 Minutes | Servings: 36 Mini Muffins

Calories: 43kcal

Ingredients

Grinch Muffins

- 1 1/2 cups white whole wheat flour (all-purpose, whole wheat pastry flour or unbleached flour also work)
- 1 tsp cinnamon
- 1 1/2 tsp baking powder
- 1/2 tsp baking soda
- 1/2 tsp salt
- 2-3 cups spinach, packed

- 3/4 cup milk, regular whole milk or a plain plant-based milk
- 1/2 cup applesauce or Happy Family Organics baby food pouch (see notes)
- 1/4 cup coconut oil, melted
- 1 ripe banana
- 1 large egg
- 1 tsp vanilla extract

Grinch Hearts

- 1/2 cup raspberries
- 3 tbsp cream cheese

Instructions

1. **Prep:** Preheat the oven to 350° F. Line a mini muffin tray with liners or grease.
2. **Dry Ingredients:** In a medium bowl, whisk together the flour, cinnamon, baking powder, baking soda and salt. Set aside.
3. **Wet Ingredients:** In a blender, add in the spinach, milk, applesauce or baby food puree, coconut oil, banana, egg and vanilla extract and blend on

medium speed for 1 minute or until all of the spinach is completely broken down, scraping sides of the blender as needed.

4. **Combine:** Pour the wet ingredients into the medium bowl of dry ingredients and gently mix together until just combined, do not over mix.

5. **Bake:** Fill the muffin molds 3/4 way full, and bake for 12-15 minutes or until they are just golden brown. Let cool completely on a wire baking rack.

6. **Prep Frosting:** To add the Grinch Hearts – spoon the cream cheese into a piping bag or a small zip lock baggie (that is what i used above). Use a rubber band to secure the top of the baggie and then cut the very corner of the baggie off to create a hole for the cream cheese to come out of.

7. **Prep "Hearts":** On a cutting board, gently cut the raspberries in half lengthwise. Then place one half of the raspberry on the cutting board, outside-facing down, and cut a small V into the top of the raspberry to make a heart shape. Place the cut side

of the raspberry onto a paper towel or kitchen towel to soak up any moisture.

8. **Decorate:** With the piping bag, on the top of the muffin make a quarter size circle of cream cheese. Then add one raspberry heart on top. Repeat until all of the muffins are decorated.

Notes

Age: for baby-led weaning 6 months and up (remove the raspberry before serving) or babies 9 months and up.

Applesauce or Baby Food Pouch: you can use either plain applesauce or for more fun flavor you can use 1/2 cup of Happy Family Organics Apple, Kale & Avocado or Spinach, Apples & Kale baby food pouch.

Storage: I recommend storing the decorated muffins in an air-tighter container in the fridge for up to 5 days. Non-decorated muffins can be stored on the counter in a slightly open container for 3 days.

Freezer-Friendly: you can freeze any non-decorated muffins for up to 3 months.

Regular Size Muffins: this recipe would work great for normal size muffins as well. Fill regular size muffin molds 3/4 the way full and bake for 20-22 minutes.

Making the Muffins Gluten-Free: You can easily makes these mini muffins gluten-free by using a cup-for-cup gluten-free flour blend.

Broccoli Egg Cups

Handheld and portable, these egg cups are great for baby and toddlers on-the-go. These savory cheddar cheese and broccoli breakfast cups can be served warm at the breakfast table or packed cold for a morning playdate or school lunch.

Course: Breakfast | Cuisine: American

Prep Time: 5 Minutes | Cook Time: 20 Minutes

Servings: 8 Egg Cups | Calories: 81kcal

Ingredients

- 6 large eggs
- 1/4 cup milk (cow, almond, coconut, hemp, etc)
- 1/2 cup broccoli chopped
- 1/2 cup cheddar cheese shredded
- salt and pepper to taste (optional)

Instructions

1. Heat oven to 375 degrees. Line 8 muffin tins with silicon muffin molds or generously spray to prevent sticking.

2. In a medium bowl, whisk the eggs and milk together.
3. Add in the broccoli, cheese, salt and pepper and stir until combined.
4. Pour the egg mixture into the muffin tins until 3/4 the way full.
5. Bake for 20-25 minutes or until eggs have set and the cheese is golden brown.

Notes

Age: 6+ months

Storage: in an air-tight container in the fridge for up to 5 days or in the freezer for up to 2 months.

Reheat Frozen: to reheat the frozen egg cups, simply place on a microwave safe plate and microwave in 30 second intervals until warm.

Avocado Toast with Hard Boiled Egg

A toddler version of the latest food sensation – Avocado Toast. The perfect quick breakfast for any modern parent and their toddler.

Course: Breakfast | Cuisine: Baby Food

Prep Time: 4 Minutes | Servings: 1 Serving

Calories: 242kcal

Ingredients

- 1 large piece of whole wheat bread (see notes below)
- 1/3 avocado, ripe
- 1 hard boiled egg, peeled

Instructions

1. Lightly toast bread.
2. Smash the avocado with the back of a fork, spread onto the toasted bread.
3. Roughly chop the hard boiled egg, sprinkle of top of avocado.

4. Cut avocado toast into strips or chunks, and serve.

Notes

Make it with Tot: This recipe is also a great one to have your toddler help you make. Ways toddler can help: load the toaster up with the bread smash the peeled avocado with the back of a fork chop the hardboiled egg with a dull kid-friendly knife spread the smashed avocado onto the toasted (and cooled) bread sprinkle the egg chunks on top of the avocado

Make it for you as well: This avocado toast is a great breakfast, or snack, for you as well. Make it the same way as the Tot version, but add red pepper flakes, Everything Bagel spice mix or a drizzle of Sirrachia on top before eating.

Note on Bread: I used a piece of whole wheat bread for this recipe, but you can use any bread your family prefers – thick cut loaf, sourdough, white, multi-grain, gluten-free.

Yield: makes 1 serving

Age: 9+ months

Almond Butter + Banana with Hemp Seed Sprinkles

A fun, and super trendy, way for toddler to have a wholesome and flavorful meal in the morning.

Course: Breakfast | Cuisine: American

Prep Time: 4 Minutes | Servings: 1 Serving

Calories: 175kcal

Ingredients

- 1 slice whole wheat or multi-grain bread
- 1/2 tbsp almond butter
- 1/2 banana, thinly sliced
- 1 tsp hemp seeds

Instructions

1. Lightly toast bread. Spread the bread with almond butter and then layer the banana slices on top.
2. Sprinkle with hemp seeds and gently cut into triangles or quarters.

Notes

Nut Butters: you can use any nut or seed butter you prefer in this recipe – peanut, cashew, sunflower, etc.

Age: 9+ months. For allergy concerns, I would recommend trying almond butter in a smaller amount before serving this toast.

Wholesome Blueberry Sheet Pan Pancakes

Sheet pan pancakes are made for parents who love to make homemade pancakes but don't love all the time standing around the stove.

Course: Breakfast | Cuisine: American

Prep Time: 5 Minutes | Cook Time: 15 Minutes

Servings: 15 Servings | Calories: 95kcal

Ingredients

- 2 cups white whole wheat flour see notes
- 1 tbsp baking powder
- 1 tsp cinnamon
- 1/4 tsp salt
- 1 cup milk (cow, almond, soy, hemp, etc)
- 1/2 cup applesauce
- 2 large eggs
- 2 tbsp olive oil or melted coconut oil
- 1 tsp vanilla extract
- 1/2 cup blueberries

Instructions

1. Preheat oven to 425 degrees. Line a 10×15 sheet pan or 9×13 baking pan with parchment paper and spray well.
2. In a medium bowl, mix together the flour, baking powder, cinnamon and salt.
3. In a another medium bowl, whisk together the milk, applesauce, eggs, oil and vanilla extract.
4. Add the wet ingredients to the dry ingredients and mix until just incorporated.
5. Pour the pancake batter onto the sheet pan and sprinkle the blueberries on top.
6. Bake for 13-15 minutes or until just browned. Let cool slightly and then cut into bars.

Notes

Age: 9+ months

Flour: you can also use 1 cup of whole wheat flour and 1 cup of white wheat or all-purpose flour.

Fruit Add-Ins: feel free too add in any chopped fruit your family prefers – strawberries, blackberries, apples, raspberries or even pineapple.

Freezer-Friendly: if you have any extras, you can place the cut pancakes into a freezer safe zip-lock baggie or stasher bag and freeze. To reheat, simply microwave for 20 second increments until just warm.

Easy Cheesy Egg Roll-Ups

These egg roll-ups are perfect for babies that are just learning to self feed. Once rolled, these cheesy eggs are firm enough for baby to hold onto, yet soft enough for baby with or without teeth to eat.

Course: Breakfast | Cuisine: American

Prep Time: 2 Minutes | Cook Time: 4 Minutes

Servings: 2 Egg Roll-Ups | Calories: 115kcal

Ingredients

- 2 eggs
- 1 tbsp milk
- 2 tbsp cheddar cheese shredded
- 1 tsp oil butter or spray

Instructions

1. Pre-heat a small non-stick pan over medium-low heat. Spray the skillet or grease with 1/2 teaspoon of oil or butter.
2. In a small bowl, whisk the eggs and milk together.

3. Spoon half of the egg mixture into the pan and cook for 2 minutes.
4. Sprinkle the cheese on top of the eggs, cover the pan with a lid, and cook for 2 more minutes.
5. Using a spatula, carefully slid the flat egg onto a cutting board. Let cool slightly for 1-2 minutes but no more or the egg will be too cool to roll.
6. Starting on one side of the egg disc, start rolling the egg as tightly as you can until completely rolled up. Place seam side down and let cool slightly. As it cools, the egg roll-up will hold it's shape.
7. Repeat cooking process with remaining egg mixture.

Notes

Age: 9+ months

Add-Ins: you can add in 1 tablespoon of any finely chopped veggie or herbs you prefer to the egg mixture before cooking.

Whole Grain Pumpkin Waffle Dippers

These freezer-friendly waffle dippers are a fun and delicious way for baby to be able to eat, as well as play with, their breakfast.

Course: Breakfast | Cuisine: American

Prep Time: 5 Minutes | Cook Time: 15 Minutes

Servings: 6 Large Waffles | Calories: 180kcal

Ingredients

Pumpkin Dippers

- 2 cups white whole wheat flour
- 1 tbsp baking powder
- 2 tsp pumpkin pie spice mix
- 1/4 tsp salt
- 1/2 cup pumpkin puree
- 2 large eggs
- 1/4 cup coconut oil melted
- 2 tbsp applesauce
- 1/2 tsp vanilla extract

- 1 1/2 cups milk of choice (cow, almond, soy, coconut, etc)

Dipping Yogurt

- 3/4 cup plain whole-fat yogurt
- 2 tbsp maple syrup
- 1/2 tsp pumpkin pie spice

Instructions

1. Heat a waffle iron on medium.
2. In a large bowl, whisk together the flour, baking powder, pumpkin pie spice and salt.
3. In a medium bowl, whisk together the pumpkin puree, eggs, coconut oil, applesauce, vanilla and milk.
4. Pour the wet ingredients into the dry ingredients and whisk until smooth. If your batter is too thick, add more milk in 1/4 cup increments until the batter resembles cake batter.
5. Pour 1/2 cup of waffle batter onto each waffle mold and cook according to your waffle irons directions.

6. To make yogurt dip, mix the yogurt with the maple syrup until well mixed. Spoon into small bowls and sprinkle with pumpkin pie spice mix.
7. Let cool slightly, cut into sticks and serve with a small bowl of the yogurt dip, applesauce or maple syrup.

Notes

Age: 9+ months and up

Freezer-Friendly: these waffles are extremely freezer friendly! Simply freeze any leftovers you have and then pop them in the toaster (if left in a full waffle shape) or into the microwave for 30-45 seconds to re-heat.

Golden Milk Waffles for Baby + Toddlers + Kids

These Golden Milk Waffles are fluffy, warming and completely ridiculously delicious, so much so that the entire family will love them! Freezer-friendly for those busy mornings on-the-go!

Course: Breakfast | Cuisine: American

Prep Time: 10 Minutes | Cook Time: 20 Minutes

Total Time: 30 Minutes | Calories: 148kcal

Ingredients

- 2 c white whole wheat flour or 1-for-1 gluten-free flour
- 1 tbsp baking powder
- 1/4 tsp salt
- 3 tsp turmeric see below for more info
- 1 tsp cinnamon
- 1/2 tsp ginger powder
- 1 pinch cardamom
- 2 large eggs
- 6 tbsp olive oil or butter

- 2 tbsp maple syrup
- 2 c milk cow, nut, coconut, hemp, etc.
- 1 tsp vanilla

Instructions

1. Heat a waffle iron on medium.
2. In a large bowl, whisk together the flour, baking powder, salt, turmeric, cinnamon, ginger and cardamom.
3. In a medium bowl, whisk together the eggs, coconut oil, maple syrup, milk and vanilla.
4. Pour the wet ingredients into the dry ingredients and whisk until smooth.
5. Pour 1/4 cup of waffle batter onto each waffle mold and cook according to your waffle irons directions.
6. Let cool slightly and serve.

Notes

Spices for Baby – You may want to reduce the quantities of the spices above if your baby is 9 months and under or if your kiddo hasn't had the chance to taste the bold flavors of turmeric, ginger and cardamom before. The quantities I would recommend reducing to are as follows: 2 tsp turmeric, 1 tsp cinnamon, 1/4 tsp ginger powder, pinch of cardamom.

Freeze and Reheat – you can absolutely freeze any leftovers waffles. To reheat simply pop a frozen waffle into the toaster or toaster oven and toast until warm.

Easy Blender Spinach Pancakes for Baby + Toddler (Allergy Friendly!)

These Easy Blender Spinach Pancakes are a great way to get spinach into baby and toddler.

Course: Breakfast | Cuisine: American

Prep Time: 5 Minutes | Cook Time: 10 Minutes

Total Time: 15 Minutes | Servings: 10 Small Pancakes

Calories: 91kcal

Ingredients

- 1 cup old-fashioned oats (use gluten-free oats if needed)
- 1 cup spinach, packed
- 1 ripe banana
- 1 egg or flax egg
- 1/2 cup milk of choice – regular, coconut, almond, hemp, etc
- 2 tablespoon oil – coconut or olive
- 1 teaspoon cinnamon

- 1 teaspoon vanilla extract
- 1 teaspoon baking powder
- 1/4 teaspoon salt

Instructions

1. In a blender, place the oats and pulse on medium speed for 30 seconds or until oats are a chunky flour consistency. You will blend them all the way up in the next step, so the oats don't have to be perfectly even right now.
2. Add in the spinach, banana, egg, milk, oil, cinnamon and vanilla extract and blend on high for 30-60 seconds or until batter is completely smooth and the spinach is completely broken down, scraping down the sides of the blender if needed.
3. Add in the baking powder and salt and blend on low for 20 seconds.
4. Heat a non-stick pan or pancake griddle over medium to medium-low heat. Pour 1/4 cup of batter onto the pan and cook for 2-3 minutes or until tiny bubbles appear on the outside of the

pancake. Flip and cook for an additional 2 minutes. If batter gets too thick, add in a tablespoon at a time of milk and re-blend until you have the right consistency.

5. Transfer pancakes to a cooling rack and repeat the process until you have used all of the batter.

Notes

Age: 6 months and up

Yield: 10 small pancakes

Freezer-Friendly: store any extra pancakes in the fridge for 1 week or in the freezer for up to 2 months. To re-heat, simply place the frozen pancake in the microwave for 30 seconds or pop them straight into the toaster.

Blender Muffin Recipes

These 3 Fall Blender Muffin Recipes are beyond moist, tender, and taste and maybe most importantly, super easy to make! It takes just five minutes of prep to make these healthy mini muffins for your toddler and kids.

Course: Dessert, Snack | Cuisine: American

Diet: Vegetarian | Prep Time: 5 Minutes

Cook Time: 13 Minutes | Total Time: 18 Minutes

Servings: 16 Mini Muffins | Calories: 42kcal

Ingredients

Pumpkin Spice Muffins for Baby + Toddler

- 1 cup dry old-fashioned oats
- 1 ripe banana
- 1/4 cup pumpkin puree
- 1 egg
- 3 tablespoons maple syrup
- 1 teaspoon cinnamon
- 1/4 teaspoon nutmeg

- 1/4 teaspoon allspice
- 1/2 teaspoon baking soda
- 1/4 teaspoon salt

Cranberry Yogurt Muffins for Baby + Toddler

- 1 cup dry old-fashioned oats
- 1 ripe banana
- 1/4 cup plain Greek yogurt
- 1 egg
- 3 tablespoons maple syrup
- 1/2 teaspoon vanilla extract
- 1/2 teaspoon baking soda
- 1/4 teaspoon salt
- 1/2 cup frozen cranberries roughly chopped
- 1 teaspoon orange zest

Apple Cinnamon Muffins for Baby + Toddler

- 1 cup dry old-fashioned oats
- 1 ripe banana
- 1/4 cup applesauce sugar-free
- 1 egg
- 3 tablespoons maple syrup

- 2 teaspoons cinnamon
- 1/2 teaspoon baking soda
- 1/4 teaspoon salt
- 1/3 cup apple peeled and finely chopped

Instructions

Pumpkin Spice Muffins for Baby + Toddler

1. Preheat oven to 350 degrees F. Spray or line a mini muffin tray.
2. In a blender, add in the oats, banana, pumpkin puree, egg, maple syrup, cinnamon, nutmeg and allspice. Blend for 20 seconds on low, scrape down the sides of the blender. Blend on high for 1-2 minutes or until all of the oats are completely broken down.
3. Add in the baking soda and salt and blend on low for 20 seconds.
4. Spoon the muffin batter out of the blender and fill the muffin tin 2/3 the way full. This scoop works great for mini muffins.

5. Bake for 8-10 minutes or until golden brown on top. Let cool and then serve.

Cranberry Yogurt Muffins for Baby + Toddler

1. Preheat oven to 350 degrees F. Spray or line a mini muffin tray.
2. In a blender, add in the oats, banana, yogurt, egg, maple syrup and vanilla extract. Blend for 20 seconds on low, scrape down the sides of the blender. Blend on high for 1-2 minutes or until all of the oats are completely broken down.
3. Add in the baking soda and salt and blend on low for 20 seconds. Add in the cranberries and orange zest and mix by hand with a spoon.
4. Spoon the muffin batter out of the blender and fill the muffin tin 2/3 the way full. This scoop works great for mini muffins.
5. Bake for 8-10 minutes or until golden brown on top. Let cool and then serve.

Apple Cinnamon Muffins for Baby + Toddler

1. Preheat oven to 350 degrees F. Spray or line a mini muffin tray.
2. In a blender, add in the oats, banana, applesauce, egg, maple syrup and cinnamon. Blend for 20 seconds on low, scrape down the sides of the blender. Blend on high for 1-2 minutes or until all of the oats are completely broken down.
3. Add in the baking soda and salt and blend on low for 20 seconds.
4. Add in the apple chunks and mix by hand.
5. Spoon the muffin batter out of the blender and fill the muffin tin 2/3 the way full.
6. Bake for 8-10 minutes or until golden brown on top. Let cool and then serve.

Notes

Age – great for 7+ months of age

Storage – in airtight container for 5 days or 3 months in freezer. These muffins are super moist and are actually better if you leave the container lid cracked.

Spiced Blender Pancakes

These spiced pancakes are gluten-free, refined sugar-free and dairy-free and are filled instead with wholesome oats, one banana, a splash of almond milk and a big pinch of warming spices. The best part – they are 100% made in a blender and the prep time is under 4 minutes!

Course: Breakfast | Cuisine: American

Prep Time: 5 Minutes | Cook Time: 10 Minutes

Servings: 7 4" Pancakes | Calories: 112kcal

Ingredients

- 1 cup dry old-fashion oats see notes
- 1 ripe banana
- 1 large egg
- 1/2 cup almond milk or milk of choice
- 1 teaspoon vanilla extract
- 1 1/2 teaspoons cinnamon
- 1/2 teaspoon dried ginger
- 1/4 teaspoon nutmeg
- 1/4 teaspoon allspice

- 1 teaspoon baking powder

Instructions

1. In a high speed blender, add in the oats, banana, eggs, milk, vanilla extract, cinnamon, ginger, nutmeg and allspice. Blend on low for 10 seconds, scrape down sides, and then blend on high for 1-2 minutes or until the oats are complete broken down and the batter is smooth. Add in the baking powder and then blend on low for 20 seconds.
2. Heat a skillet on medium heat and spray with cooking spray, olive oil or coconut oil. Pour roughly 1/4 cup of pancake batter onto skillet and cook until bubbles appear, flip and cook for 2 more minutes. Continue process until all the batter is gone.
3. I find that sometimes the batter gets a little too thick during the waiting process. If that happens, add a tablespoon of milk into the batter at a time, and blend until you have the right consistency.

Notes

- If gluten free, make sure you use oats that are specified as Gluten Free.
- Store in air-tight container in fridge for 1 week or freezer for 2 months. Reheat frozen pancakes in the microwave for 20-30 seconds or by popping them into your toaster.
- **Age:** great for babies 7+ months of age, toddler and even adults

4 Baked Oatmeal Cups for Baby, Toddler + Kids

These allergy-friendly Baked Oatmeal Cups are about to make your crazy mornings a whole lot easier (and more delicious)!

Course: Breakfast | Cuisine: American

Prep Time: 10 Minutes | Cook Time: 30 Minutes

Servings: 12 Oat Muffins | Calories: 256kcal

Ingredients

Base of Oatmeal Cups

- 3 cups old fashioned oats, separated (see instructions)
- 2 tsp baking powder
- 1 tsp cinnamon
- 1/2 tsp salt
- 2 large ripe bananas, smashed (roughly 1 cup)
- 2 eggs
- 1 cup almond milk, or milk of choice
- 1/4 cup maple syrup
- 1/4 cup coconut oil melted

- 2 tsp vanilla extract

Carrot Cake Add-Ins

- 1/2 cup carrots, shredded
- 1/4 cup raisins (I used the golden variety)
- 1/4 tsp nutmeg

Antioxidant Powerhouse

- 2 cups frozen raspberries, roughly chopped
- 1/4 cup mini dark chocolate chips (optional)
- 1 tbsp chia seeds

PB&J

- 1/2 cup peanut butter, or any nutbutter
- 1/4 cup jam

Almond Blueberry

- 1/2 cup fresh or frozen blueberries
- 1/4 cup slivered almonds
- 1 tsp almond extract

Instructions

1. Preheat oven to 350 degrees F. Line or spray 12 muffin tins.
2. Take 1 cup of the old fashioned oats and pour into a blender or food processor. Pulse the oats for 30 seconds or until you they resemble a thick flour that resembles corn flour. Don't over pulse or you will get a sticky flour. You can also use 1 cup of pre-made oat flour instead of grinding your own.
3. In a large bowl, whisk together the oats, oat flour, baking powder, cinnamon and salt.
4. In a medium bowl, whisk together the smashed bananas, eggs, milk, syrup, coconut oil and vanilla extract.
5. Pour the wet ingredients into the dry ingredients and stir until incorporated.
6. Gently stir in add-ins.
7. Spoon oat batter into the muffins tins all the way to the top.
8. Bake for 30 minutes or until just golden brown on top. Let cool slightly and serve.

Notes

Note on Oats: if making gluten free, make sure your oats are labeled gluten free. Here is our favorite brand of gluten free old-fashioned oats.

Age: 6 months and up if doing baby-led weaning. Great for toddlers and kids as well.

Note on Baby-Led Weaning: If serving to baby under 1 year of age, you can skip the maple syrup. I would recommend startig baby with the base recipe and then adding in finely chopped toppings as you see fit.

Yield: 12 Oat Cups

Storage: in an air-tight container in the fridge for 5 days. These muffins freeze wonderfully. Simply place the oat cups in a freezer bag, press out any excess air, seal and freeze for up to 3 months. To reheat, simply place the frozen oat cups in the microwave for 30-60 seconds or until unfrozen and slightly warm.

Note on Chocolate: if making these dairy-free, make sure you sue dairy-free chocolate. This is our favorite brand.

Sweet Potato Waffles for Baby and Toddler

These mini sweet potato waffles are perfect for baby's first finger foods – easy to grasp, easy to gnaw on and easy for you to enjoy right along with them!

Course: Main Course | Cuisine: American

Prep Time: 10 Minutes | Cook Time: 15 Minutes

Servings: 12 Toddler Size

Ingredients

- 1 1/2 cups whole wheat, white whole wheat or all-purpose flour
- 1 cup quick oats
- 3 tsp baking powder
- 1 tsp cinnamon
- 1/4 tsp salt
- 2 eggs
- 1 cup whole milk
- 1/2 cup plain whole fat yogurt
- 3 tbsp coconut oil or butter

- 4 ounces sweet potato puree homemade or store bought
- 2 tbsp brown sugar or maple syrup

Instructions

1. In a large bowl, whisk together the flour, oats, baking powder, cinnamon, and salt until combined.
2. Whisk in the eggs, milk, yogurt, oil, puree and brown sugar into the flour mixture until all ingredients are combined. Let stand for 10 minutes while you pre-heat your waffle maker.
3. If your batter is too thick, add in an additional 1-2 tablespoons of milk.
4. Pour in roughly 2 tablespoons batter onto lightly greased waffle maker for baby size waffle or 1/4 cup batter for toddler size waffle. Shut lid and cook based on your waffle makers directions. Lift waffle out with fork, slightly cool. Serve or freeze.

Notes

Yield – 12 toddler size or 24 baby size waffles

Storage – 5 days in fridge or 3 months in freezer

Oats – quick oats are ideal in this recipe so the grain isn't too big for baby to chew. If you want to use old-fashion oats, give them a quick blitz in food processor so they are half the original size.

Sweet Potato Puree – You can use homemade or store bought sweet potato puree in this recipe. You can also use any puree you have on hand – apple, carrot, pumpkin, squash, peach, etc. Or sub in homemade or store bought applesauce.

Avocado + Blueberry Yummy Toddler Mini Muffins

Delicious toddler muffins made with avocado and blueberries!

Prep Time: 5 Mins | Cook Time: 25 Mins | Total Time: 30 Mins

Ingredients

- 2 cups white whole wheat flour (whole wheat, unbleached, gluten free mix also will work)
- 2 tsp baking powder
- 1/2 tsp baking soda
- 1/2 tsp salt
- 1 ripe organic avocado, seeded and peeled
- 1/2 cup sugar
- 1 egg
- 1 tsp vanilla extract
- 1/2 tsp cinnamon
- 1 cup plain whole-fat yogurt
- 1 1/4 cup blueberries

- 1/2 cup raw sugar for topping (optional)

Instructions

1. Heat oven to 375 and spray or line a regular or mini muffin tin.
2. In a medium bowl, combine the flour, baking powder, baking soda and salt.
3. In a large bowl, with a hand mixer, mix the avocado until smooth and creamy. Add in the sugar and mix well. Add in the egg, and mix until completely combined. Add in the vanilla, yogurt and cinnamon and mix well.
4. Pour in the flour mixture 1/3 at a time, mixing until just combined.
5. Gently fold in blueberries.
6. Spoon into muffin tin, filling 3/4 way to the top. Sprinkle raw sugar on top of each muffin.
7. Bake for 15 minutes for mini muffins or 25-30 minutes for regular muffins, or until toothpick domes out clean. Let cool in pan for 5 minutes before transitioning to cooling rack.

Spiced Blender Pancakes

These spiced pancakes are gluten-free, refined sugar-free and dairy-free and are filled instead with wholesome oats, one banana, a splash of almond milk and a big pinch of warming spices. The best part – they are 100% made in a blender and the prep time is under 4 minutes!

Course: Breakfast | Cuisine: American

Prep Time: 5 Minutes | Cook Time: 10 Minutes

Servings: 7 4" Pancakes | Calories: 112kcal

Ingredients

- 1 cup dry old-fashion oats see notes
- 1 ripe banana
- 1 large egg
- 1/2 cup almond milk or milk of choice
- 1 teaspoon vanilla extract
- 1 1/2 teaspoons cinnamon
- 1/2 teaspoon dried ginger
- 1/4 teaspoon nutmeg
- 1/4 teaspoon allspice

- 1 teaspoon baking powder

Instructions

1. In a high speed blender, add in the oats, banana, eggs, milk, vanilla extract, cinnamon, ginger, nutmeg and allspice. Blend on low for 10 seconds, scrape down sides, and then blend on high for 1-2 minutes or until the oats are complete broken down and the batter is smooth. Add in the baking powder and then blend on low for 20 seconds.
2. Heat a skillet on medium heat and spray with cooking spray, olive oil or coconut oil. Pour roughly 1/4 cup of pancake batter onto skillet and cook until bubbles appear, flip and cook for 2 more minutes. Continue process until all the batter is gone.
3. I find that sometimes the batter gets a little too thick during the waiting process. If that happens, add a tablespoon of milk into the batter at a time, and blend until you have the right consistency.

Notes

If gluten free, make sure you use oats that are specified as Gluten Free.

Store in air-tight container in fridge for 1 week or freezer for 2 months. Reheat frozen pancakes in the microwave for 20-30 seconds or by popping them into your toaster.

Age: great for babies 7+ months of age, toddler and even adults

Lunch Recipes

Cheesy Broccoli Quinoa Bites

This handheld meal is a fun way to serve broccoli to your toddler.

Course: Main Course | Cuisine: American

Prep Time: 5 Minutes | Cook Time: 22 Minutes

Servings: 12 Mini Muffins

Ingredients

- 1 cup cooked quinoa
- 1/2 cup cheddar cheese shredded
- 1/2 cup broccoli finely chopped
- 1 large egg
- 1/2 teaspoon garlic powder
- 1/4 teaspoon onion powder

Instructions

1. Preheat oven to 350 degrees. Spray or line a mini-muffin pan.
2. In a medium bowl, mix all the ingredients together.

3. Fill each muffin cup by dropping in two tablespoons of the quinoa mixture into each muffin cup, pressing down the mixture.
4. Bake for 20-22 minutes or until golden brown on top.
5. Let cool slightly and serve.

Notes

Servings: Makes 12 mini muffins

Age: 9+ months

Mini Bagel Pizzas with Pepper "Sprinkles"

These easy-peasy pizzas come with a fun surprise – pepper "sprinkles". Toddlers will love adding these bright and colorful veggie sprinkles onto their lunch pizzas.

Course: Main Course | Cuisine: American

Prep Time: 5 Minutes | Cook Time: 10 Minutes

Servings: 2 2 Bagel Serving

Ingredients

- 2 mini whole grain bagels cut in half
- 1/3 cup marinara sauce
- 1/2 cup mozzarella cheese shredded
- 1/4 cup chopped peppers red, yellow, orange and/or green

Instructions

1. Heat oven to 425 degrees. Place tin foil on a baking sheet for easy clean up.
2. Top each half of a bagel with the marinara sauce, spreading all the way to the edge.

3. Top with roughly 2 tablespoons of mozzarella.
4. Sprinkle on the peppers.
5. Place on baking sheet and bake for 8-10 minutes or until the cheese is melted and bubbly.
6. Let cool and serve

Notes

Serving: 2 servings of 2 bagel pizzas each

Age: 12+ Months

Tortellini On-a-Stick with Marinara Dipping Sauce

Your toddler will flip-out with excitement when you serve them their lunch on-a-stick! This easy lunch is made with leftover tortellini and any chopped veggies your toddler prefers.

Course: Main Course | Cuisine: American

Prep Time: 5 Minutes

Ingredients

- 1/2 cup tortellini cooked and cooled
- 1/4 cup cherry tomatoes
- 1/4 cup black olives
- 1/4 cup mushrooms quartered
- 1/2 cup marinara sauce
- 6-8 wooden skewers

Instructions

1. Cut cherry tomatoes and black olives in half, if needed.

2. Take a wooden skewer and thread on all the ingredients in any order you prefer.
3. Heat the marinara sauce up in microwave for 30 seconds or in a small pot on the stove.

Notes

Wooden Skewer: you can use any wooden skewer you have on hand, but make sure to cut the pointy end off before serving. I use wooden coffee stir sticks when I serve this recipe.

Time-Saving Tip: use leftover tortellini in this recipe to save on prep-time.

Veggie Tip: feel free to use any veggies that your toddler loves in this recipe – chunks of peppers, broccoli florets, cauliflower florets, etc.

Age: 12 + Months

Curry Pasta Salad for Baby + Toddler

Bite sized pasta, broccoli, carrots and chickpeas get tossed in a tasty mild curry sauce that will delight any baby or toddler's growing taste buds! This finger food salad is a fun way to introduce curry to baby. Perfect for baby-led weaning and the finger food stage!

Course: Main Course | Cuisine: Indian

Prep Time: 10 Minutes | Cook Time: 10 Minutes

Total Time: 20 Minutes | Servings: 4

Ingredients

Pasta Salad

- 1 cup dry pasta small to medium shaped pasta works best
- 1/3 cup carrots peeled and finely chopped
- 1/3 cup broccoli finely chopped
- 1/3 cup chick peas skins removed and cut in half

Curry Dressing

- 1/4 cup plain yogurt
- 1/2 tbsp apple cider vinegar
- 1/2 tbsp olive oil
- 1/2 tsp agave nectar optional
- 1/2 tsp mild curry powder
- 1/4 tsp turmeric powder
- 1/4 tsp garlic powder
- 1/4 tsp ginger powder or 1/8 tsp freshly grated ginger
- pinch pink Himalayan salt

Instructions

1. In a medium saucepan, cook pasta according to directions on package. When you have 2 minutes left on the timer, add in the chopped carrots, broccoli and chick peas and let cook for the remaining time.
2. Drain pasta, carrots, broccoli and chick peas and let cool slightly.

3. Meanwhile, in a small bowl, add the yogurt, apple cider vinegar, olive oil, agave nectar (if using), curry, turmeric, garlic, ginger and salt and mix well.
4. Transfer the pasta, carrots, broccoli and chick peas to a medium bowl.
5. Add in the curry dressing 1 tablespoon at a time until you have your desired sauce-to-pasta ratio. You will probably not use the entire batch of curry dressing. I used a little over 2 tablespoons in the recipe above. You can save the rest of the curry dressing. I love using my left over curry dressing as a dip for my kids alongside an assortment offresh or roasted veggies.
6. Serve and enjoy.

Notes

Other Fun Foods to Add to this Pasta Salad

- 1/2 cup chicken, cooked and chopped/shredded
- 1/4 cup celery, chopped
- 1/3 cup zucchini, chopped (cook in pasta water)
- 1/4 cup golden raisins, chopped (for toddlers)

- 2 tablespoons parsley, freshly chopped

Summer Pesto Finger Salad for Baby + Toddler

This Pesto Summer Finger Salad for Baby + Toddler is full of bite-size pieces of corn, tomatoes, zucchini and orzo pasta all mixed together with a spoonful of flavorful pesto. This finger salad is a great way for baby to enjoy the delicious tastes of summer.

Course: Baby Led Weaning | Cuisine: American

Ingredients

- 1/2 cup dry orzo pasta
- 1/4 cup zucchini finely chopped
- 1/4 cup corn
- 1/4 cup tomatoes deseeded and finely chopped
- 2 tablespoons pesto homemade or store-bought

Instructions

1. Fill a medium saucepan 3/4 of the way with water, bring to a boil over high heat. Add in the orzo and cook for 6 minutes. Add in the corn and zucchini and cook for 1 more additional minute.

2. Drain pasta and veggies in a colander and rinse with cold water. Let cool to touch.
3. Transfer pasta and veggies to a medium bowl or storage container with lid. Add in pesto and tomatoes, mix until combined. Serve cold or slightly warmed.

Notes

Note on Corn - freshly cut kernels from the cob work best but you can also used canned or frozen.

Green Finger Salad for Baby + Toddler

Gently steamed green veggies are tossed in coconut oil and a pinch of fresh mint for a taste-sensation. Great for baby-led weaning or the finger food stage.

Course: Main Course | Cuisine: Baby Food

Prep Time: 5 Minutes | Cook Time: 15 Minutes

Servings: 2 Cups

Ingredients

- 1/2 cup asparagus, trimmed and chopped
- 1/2 cup green beans, trimmed and chopped
- 1 cup broccoli florets, chopped
- 1/2 tsp coconut oil
- 3 mint sprigs, finely chopped

Instructions

Nutribaby

1. Place the asparagus, green beans and broccoli into the large basket. Start the steam cycle for 8 minutes. Let cool slightly.

2. Place all of the ingredients into a medium bowl, and toss with the coconut oil and mint. The coconut oil will melt as you toss the warm veggies in it.

Regular Cooking Method

1. In a medium saucepan, bring 2 inches of water to a boil. Add the asparagus, green beans and broccoli into a steamer basket, cover and steam for 8 minutes. Let cool slightly.
2. Transfer all ingredients into a medium bowl, and toss with the coconut oil and mint.

Notes

Age: 6+ months

Yield: 2 cups or 6 small servings

Storage: Fridge – store in an airtight container in the fridge for 4-5 days.

Snacks Recipes

Veggie-Loaded Hummus for Baby and Toddler

This Veggie-Loaded Hummus Baby Food or Toddler Dip is an amazing recipe that grows with your baby!

Course: Main Course | Cuisine: Baby Food

Prep Time: 5 Minutes | Cook Time: 20 Minutes

Total Time: 25 Minutes | Servings: 18 Ounces, 2 Cups Of Dip

Ingredients

For Baby Puree

- 3 medium carrots, peeled and roughly chopped
- 1 small sweet potato, peeled and roughly chopped (roughly 1 cup)
- 1/4 cup canned chickpeas, drained and rinsed

For Toddler Dip

- 3 medium carrots, peeled and roughly chopped
- 1 small sweet potato, peeled and roughly chopped

- 1 cup canned chickpeas, drained and rinsed
- 1 clove garlic
- 1 tsp cumin or mild curry powder
- 2 tbsp olive oil
- 1/2 tsp salt

Instructions

1. In a medium saucepan, bring 2 inches of water to a boil. In a steamer basket, add in the sweet potato cubes and carrots, place basket over boiling water and cover. Steam for 12-15 minutes or until all ingredients are tender when pricked with a fork. Remove from heat and let cool slightly. Reserve steamer water.

To Make For Baby

1. Transfer the cooked carrots, sweet potato as well as the chickpeas into a blender or food processor.
2. Puree for 2 minutes or until smooth, adding in additional reserved steamer water in 1/4 cup increments if needed.

To Make for Toddler

1. Transfer the cooked carrots, sweet potato, chickpeas, garlic, cumin or mild curry powder, olive oil and salt into a food processor.
2. Puree for 1-2 minutes or until smooth adding in additional water, reserved water or olive oil in 1/4 cup increments if needed.

Notes

To make this for a baby as well as a toddler: follow directions as stated above for the baby puree. Once you have baby's portion blended, remove roughly one cup of the puree and set aside for baby. Add in the toddler ingredients to the blender or food processor (this recipe is very verstile so if you add in a few more chickpeans this way, then you will just get a thicker hummus) and blend until smooth.

Spice it Up for Toddler: To spice up the toddler version even more, feel free to add in 2 tbsp tahini, 1/2 juiced lemon and/or 1/4 tsp paprika.

Spice it Up for Baby: To spice it up for baby, you can add in 1/4 tsp cumin or mild curry powder to their puree.

Yield: 18 ounces of puree, 2 cups of dip

Age: 7+ months and up

Warm Peach Chunks with Nutmeg for Baby & Toddler

Warmed chunks of peaches pair perfectly with a pinch of nutmeg for a naturally sweetened finger food for baby. You can serve the peach chunks by themselves or add them to the top of yogurt, cottage cheese or smeared on top of a piece of toast to use instead of jam.

Course: Breakfast, Dessert, Snack | Cuisine: Baby Food, Toddler Food | Cook Time: 10 Minutes

Total Time: 10 Minutes | Servings: 6 Servings

Ingredients

- 2 cups peaches peeled and sliced (fresh or frozen)
- 1/4 teaspoon nutmeg
- 1/4 teaspoon vanilla
- 2 tablespoons of water

Instructions

1. In a small saucepan, place all of the ingredients.

2. Cook on medium-low heat for 5-10 minutes or until peaches are warm and you can break them up with the back of a wooden spoon.
3. Let cool slightly, chop into finger size pieces and serve.

Notes

Age: 6+ months and up. For 6-9 months chop into "pea" size pieces or 2-3 inch long strips before serving.

Serving options: can be served plain, over yogurt or cottage cheese or smeared on top of a piece of toast instead of jam.

Storage: store in air-tight container in fridge for up to a week.

Healthy Strawberry Cream Cheese Dip

Let your toddler have their fun and eat it to! Toddlers love to dip and this naturally sweetened dip is a winner.

Course: Side Dish, Snack | Cuisine: Baby Food, Toddler Food | Cook Time: 5 Minutes | Total Time: 5 Minutes

Servings: 4 Servings

Ingredients

- 1/2 cup strawberries fresh or frozen and thawed
- 1/4 cup cream cheese
- 1/4 cup plain full-fat Greek yogurt

Instructions

1. Place all dip ingredients into a blender or food processor and pulse in 2 second intervals until strawberries are chopped and the dip is mixed.
2. Spoon dip into a air-tight container and place in the fridge for 30 minutes to harden.
3. Serve with your favorite dipping ingredients.

Notes

Dippers: Serve with an assortment of dipping items – cut strawberries, pretzels, graham crackers, fruit skewers, pineapple wedges, banana slices, kiwi chunks, berries, apple slices, etc

age: 9+ months

storage: keep in an air-tight container in the fridge for up to one week.

Easy Whole Grain Baked Cheese Crackers

These snack-able whole grain crackers are going to be a big hit with your toddler. With no rolling involved, these wholesome crackers are also a snap to make.

Course: Side Dish, Snack | Cuisine: Toddler Food

Prep Time: 5 Minutes | Cook Time: 11 Minutes

Chill Time: 45 Minutes | Total Time: 16 Minutes

Servings: 12 Servings

Ingredients

- 6 oz or 2 cups cheddar cheese shredded
- 3/4 cup whole wheat flour or white whole wheat flour
- 1/4 cup butter
- 1/2 teaspoon salt
- 1/4 teaspoon garlic powder
- 1-2 tablespoons milk or water

Instructions

1. In a food processor, place the cheese, butter, flour, salt and garlic powder and pulse until chunky.
2. Add in 1 tablespoon of liquid and turn on the food process until a dough ball forms. If ball isn't forming, add another tablespoon of liquid.
3. Dust a work surface with a little flour. Roll the dough into a ball and then divid it into 4 balls. With your hands roll each ball into a 1/2 inch rope. Wrap the 4 ropes in saran wrap and place in the freeze for 45-60 minutes or until just hard to the touch.
4. Preheat oven to 350 degrees. Spray a baking sheet with cooking spray.
5. Take out the dough ropes and slice into 1/4 inch slices. Place on baking sheet and press a dot in the middle of each cracker with a wooden skewer or a fork.
6. Bake for 11-13 minutes or just golden brown. Let cool completely on the baking sheet, they will continue to crisp up as they cool.

Notes

age: 9+ months

storage: store in a container on the counter for up to 1 week. I like to leave the container lid cracked so the crackers don't get too soggy.

Dinner Recipes

Crispy Herb Salmon Bites for Baby + Toddler

These salmon bites are a great way to introduce salmon to baby or toddler in an easy-to-eat foolproof way.

Course: Main Course | Cuisine: American

Prep Time: 10 Minutes | Cook Time: 15 Minutes

Total Time: 25 Minutes | Servings: 6 Small Servings

Ingredients

- 1/2 lb salmon fillets skin removed, cut into 1" thick pieces
- 1/4 cup white whole wheat flour
- 2 large eggs
- 1 cup Panko breadcrumbs
- 1 tablespoon Italian seasoning
- 3 teaspoons dried parsley
- salt and pepper to taste (optional)

Instructions

1. Preheat oven to 450 degree F. Spray or line a baking sheet.
2. Pat dry the salmon pieces.
3. In a small bowl, stir the flour and salt and pepper (if using) together.
4. In another small bowl, whisk the eggs together
5. In another small bowl, stir the breadcrumbs, seasoning, parsley, salt and pepper (if using) together.
6. One at a time, coat the salmon pieces. First coat the salmon in the flour, dusting off any excess, then dip in the egg mixture and then toss in the breadcrumbs until completely coated. Place coated salmon pieces onto baking sheet.
7. Bake for 15-17 minutes or until crispy and golden brown.
8. Serve with steamed broccoli and cauliflower.

Notes

Fish: you can use this recipe on any firm fish your family prefers.

Age: 9+ months

Easy Veggie "Fried" Rice for Baby + Toddler

This healthy version of the classic dish is filled with your favorite rice, a mix of veggies and a scrambled egg for some protein. You can use whichever veggies your little one prefers to make this dish and instant classic in your home.

Course: Main Course | Cuisine: Chinese

Prep Time: 5 Minutes | Cook Time: 10 Minutes

Total Time: 15 Minutes | Servings: 6 1/2 Cup Servings

Ingredients

- 1 tablespoon olive oil
- 1 cup mix of chopped vegetables fresh or frozen
- 1 clove garlic minced
- 1 egg
- 2 cups cooked rice jasmine, brown or riced cauliflower
- 1 tablespoon coconut amnios or low-sodium soy sauce
- 1 teaspoon sesame oil

Instructions

1. In a medium skillet, over medium heat, heat the oil. Add in the vegetables and garlic and sauté for 3-5 minutes or until tender.
2. Turn the heat to low, and push the vegetables to the side of the skillet. Crack the egg directly into the skillet and scramble for 3-4 minutes. Mix the egg pieces in with the vegetables.
3. Add in the cooked rice, coconut amnios and sesame oil and mix until incorporated.
4. Let cool slightly. Cut any vegetables into pea size pieces before serving.

Notes

age: 9+ months

Taco Tuesday for Baby

Don't forget about baby's dinner on your favorite meal night of the week – Taco Tuesday! This flavorful meal is filled with your favorite taco flavors, only mini-sized for those little hands to be able to eat.

Course: Main Course | Cuisine: Mexican

Prep Time: 5 Minutes | Cook Time: 15 Minutes

Total Time: 20 Minutes | Servings: 6 Small Servings

Ingredients

- 1 tablespoon olive oil
- 1/2 lb lean ground turkey
- 1/2 cup canned black beans rinsed
- 2 teaspoons chili powder
- 1 teaspoon paprika
- 1/2 teaspoon garlic powder
- 1/4 teaspoon onion powder
- 2 tablespoons water
- 1/3 cup cheese shredded

Serve With

- 1/2 avocado chopped
- 1/2 pepper chopped into strips
- 1/2 tomato finely chopped

Instructions

1. Heat olive oil in a medium pan over medium heat. Add in the turkey and cook until browned, stirring every couple of minutes to break up the bigger meat chunks.
2. Add in the beans, chili powder, paprika, garlic powder, onion powder and water and stir until combined. Turn down heat to low and simmer for 5-10 minutes, stirring occasionally.
3. Turn off heat, and let turkey mixture cool slightly. Spoon turkey and bean mixture onto a baby-friendly plate and sprinkle the cheese on top.
4. Serve with avocado chunks, pepper strips and tomato chunks or any of your favorite taco toppings.

Notes

For an adult version: serve the same ingredients inside of your favorite taco shell and top with salsa and freshly chopped cilantro.

Age: 9+ months

Mexican Sweet Potato Boats

These sweet potato boats are a family-friendly way to serve sweet potatoes to the entire family – including those picky eaters.

Course: Main Course | Cuisine: Mexican

Prep Time: 10 Minutes | Cook Time: 10 Minutes

Total Time: 20 Minutes | Servings: 6 1/2 Potato Servings

Ingredients

- 3 cooked small whole sweet potatoes
- 1/2 cup black beans
- 1/2 cup corn
- 1/4 teaspoon paprika
- 1/4 teaspoon garlic powder
- 1/4 teaspoon cumin
- 1/2 avocado chopped
- 1 small tomato finely chopped
- 1/4 cup cheddar cheese shredded
- 1 tablespoon cilantro finely chopped

Instructions

1. Warm the sweet potatoes in the microwave or in a 350 degree oven.
2. In a medium skillet, add in the black beans, corn, paprika, garlic powder and cumin and cook for 5 minutes over medium-low heat, stirring often.
3. Cut the sweet potatoes in half, using a spoon to scrap the sweet potato away from the skin and cut or smash the sweet potato into small chunks, being careful not to cut the peel.
4. Add 1/4 cup of the bean and corn mixture on top of the sweet potato.
5. Sprinkle the avocado, tomatoes, cheese and cilantro on top and serve.

Notes

Serving for Baby: You can also serve this same meal but without the sweet potato skin, which can sometimes be confusing for babies and toddlers. Simply discard the skin and put the sweet potato and toppings on a plate or in a bowl.

Age: 9+ months

Baked Seasoned Chicken Tenders

An easy and healthy sheet pan meal for baby – tender seasoned chicken tenders with a side of roasted sweet potato chunks.

Course: Drinks | Cuisine: American

Prep Time: 5 Minutes | Cook Time: 20 Minutes

Total Time: 25 Minutes | Servings: 6 Small Servings

Ingredients

Baked Chicken Tenders

- 1/2 pound chicken tenders
- 1 teaspoon olive oil
- 1/2 teaspoon paprika
- 1/2 teaspoon garlic powder
- 1/4 teaspoon onion powder

Roasted Sweet Potatoes

- 1 small sweet potato peeled and finely cubed or cut into strips
- 2 teaspoons olive oil

- 1/2 teaspoon garlic powder
- 1/2 teaspoon dried oregano

Instructions

1. Preheat oven to 450 degree F. Spray or line a baking sheet.
2. In a medium bowl, toss the cubes of sweet potatoes in the olive oil, garlic powder and oregano.
3. Place the sweet potatoes on one side of the baking sheet.
4. In the same medium bowl, toss the chicken in the olive oil, paprika, garlic powder and onion powder.
5. Place the chicken on the other side of the baking sheet.
6. Bake for 18-20 minutes or until chicken is cooked all the way through. Take out the chicken and let it rest on a cutting board.
7. Flip the sweet potatoes and cook for an additional 10-15 minutes or until tender when pricked with a fork. Let cool slightly. Cut or shred chicken into

small pieces and cut sweet potatoes into smaller pieces if needed.

Notes

Sweet Potato Options: You can also cut the sweet potato into long strips for some healthy fries for baby + toddler!

Age: 9+ months

Baked Seasoned Tofu Finger Food Nuggets

These crispy bite-sized pieces of tofu are a fun and tasty way for baby to get protein in their diet.

Course: Main Course, Side Dish, Snack

Cuisine: Baby Food | Prep Time: 30 Minutes

Cook Time: 30 Minutes | Total Time: 1 Hour

Servings: 6 Servings

Ingredients

- 1 block extra-firm tofu organic recommended
- 1 tablespoon olive oil extra virgin
- 1 tablespoon arrowroot powder
- 1/4 teaspoon garlic powder
- 1/4 teaspoon mild chili powder
- 1/4 teaspoon paprika

Instructions

1. To get the tofu crispy, you have to drain any excess water from it. Slice the block of tofu horizontally into 2 or 3 even slabs and place tofu slabs on top of

a stack of paper towels, with paper towels between each layer and on top of the top slab of tofu. Place a weight on top of the stack of tofu (books, cast iron skillet, cans, etc) and let the tofu drain for 15-30 minutes.
2. Meanwhile, heat oven to 400-degree F and spray a baking sheet.
3. Cut the tofu into cubes, strips or triangles and place into a medium bowl.
4. Drizzle with olive oil and gently toss to coat. Then sprinkle with the arrowroot powder and the remaining spices and gently toss to coat.
5. Place tofu onto baking sheet and bake for 25-30 minutes, flipping halfway through baking time.

Notes

Age: 6+ months and up. Cut into smaller chunks or 2-3 inch strips for 6-12-month olds.

Serving Suggestion – these bite-size tofu nuggets are great served warm along with your child's favorite veggie or fruit for a tasty protein packed finger food snack or meal.

Storage: store in air-tight container in fridge for up to 1 week.

Reheat: you can serve cold, or reheat in a skillet over med-low heat until just warm.

Kale Pesto Chicken Quesadilla

This baby-friendly chicken quesadilla is amped-up with a secret ingredient – kale!

Course: Main Course | Cuisine: American

Prep Time: 5 Minutes | Cook Time: 5 Minutes

Total Time: 10 Minutes | Servings: 4 2 Wedge Servings

Ingredients

- 2 small whole wheat tortillas
- 1 tablespoon kale pesto store bought or homemade
- 1/3 cup cooked chicken finely cubed or shredded
- 1/4 cup mozzarella cheese shredded

Instructions

1. Heat a large skillet over medium heat.
2. Lay the tortillas on a cutting board and spread the pesto onto one side of each tortilla.

3. Take one tortilla and sprinkle the chicken and cheese on top. Layer the other tortilla on top, pesto facing down.
4. Place tortillas onto the hot skillet and cook for 3 minutes per side or until golden brown and the cheese is melted.
5. Let cool slightly and then cut into 8 wedges.

Notes

Homemade Kale Pesto – in a food processor pulse together 1 cup packed kale, 1 cup packed basil, 1/2 lemon juiced, 2 cloves of garlic, 1/2 cup parmesan cheese, 1/2 cup oil olive, salt and pepper to taste (optional) until fully combined.

Age: 9+ months

Baby's First Bolognese

A thick and hearty bolognese sauce with added veggies is the perfect way to introduce this classic sauce to your baby. This sauce is versatile and can be served over your favorite pasta, brown rice, zucchini noodles or spaghetti squash.

Course: Main Course | Cuisine: Italian

Prep Time: 10 Minutes | Cook Time: 20 Minutes

Total Time: 30 Minutes | Servings: 6 1/2 Cup Per Serving

Ingredients

- 1/2 teaspoon olive oil
- 1/2 cup onion diced
- 1 clove garlic minced
- 1/2 pound ground turkey beef, chicken or pork
- 1 small carrot peeled and finely chopped
- 1/3 cup zucchini finely chopped
- 1-28 oz can crushed tomatoes
- 1 tablespoon tomato paste
- 1 teaspoon dried parsley
- 1/2 teaspoon dried basil

- 1/4 teaspoon dried oregano

Instructions

1. In a large skillet over medium heat, heat the olive oil. Add in the onion and garlic and let cook for 2-3 minutes or until translucent, stirring often.
2. Add in the ground meat and cook for 4-5 minutes or until browned, stirring often to break up the meat. Drain any excess fat.
3. Add in the carrot and zucchini and cook for 2-3 minutes.
4. Add in the tomatoes, tomato paste, parsley, basil and oregano and let it come to a boil.
5. Reduce heat and let simmer for 10-20 minutes.

Notes

Serve with: pasta of your choice (original, whole wheat, gluten free, lentil, chickpea), spaghetti squash, brown rice or even zucchini noodles.

Age: 9+ months and up

Easy-Peasy 5 Veggie Pasta for Baby

This wholesome baby-led weaning meal is made by tossing together your favorite pasta, a whopping 5 different veggies and a simple yet delicious basil dressing. Everything is the same finger food size for easy eating for baby.

Course: Main Course | Cuisine: American

Prep Time: 5 Minutes | Cook Time: 10 Minutes

Total Time: 15 Minutes | Servings: 6 Servings

Ingredients

- 1 cup pasta of choice original, whole wheat, gluten free, lentil, bean, etc
- 1 cup mix of chopped vegetables fresh or frozen
- 2 tablespoons olive oil
- 2 teaspoons dried basil
- 1/2 teaspoon garlic powder
- 2 tablespoons parmesan

Instructions

1. Fill a large stockpot 3/4 the way full of water, and bring to a boil. Cook pasta according to package. If using fresh vegetables – when you have 2 minutes left on the timer, add in the vegetables into the pasta water. If using frozen vegetables – when you have 4 minutes left on the timer, add in the vegetables into the pasta water.
2. Meanwhile, stir together the olive oil, garlic powder and dried basil. Set aside.
3. Drain the pasta and vegetables.
4. In the same stockpot, add in the cook pasta, vegetables and olive oil mixture. Toss to combine. Sprinkle with parmesan and serve.

Notes

Veggie Suggestion: you can use almost any veggies you have on hand for this dish – broccoli, cauliflower, peas, squash, peas, corn, green beans, asparagus, mushrooms, peppers, carrots, sweet potato, etc. The key is to chop them into small pieces so they cook in a short amount of time and so they are also easy for baby and tot to eat.

Age: 9+ months

Storage: store in air-tight container in fridge for up to 5 days. Can be served warmed in microwave or cold.

Chunky Summer Veggie Pasta

This Chunky Summer Veggie Pasta for Baby and Toddler combines all the flavorful tastes of summer into one bite-size dish!

Course: Main Course | Cuisine: Baby Food

Prep Time: 5 Minutes | Cook Time: 15 Minutes

Servings: 12 Ounces

Ingredients

- 1/2 small zucchini
- 6 asparagus spears
- 1 leek white and light green parts only
- 8-10 basil leaves
- 1/2 lemon, juiced
- 1/4 cup + 2 tbsp small shaped pasta
- 1/2 cup + 3 tbsp water
- sprinkle of parmesan, optional

Instructions

Instructions using Beaba's Babycook Pro

1. Chop the zucchini, asparagus and leek into 1" pieces. Roughly chop the basil.
2. Fill one basket with the zucchini, asparagus and leek. Using the measuring bowl, fill the correlating heating tank to a level 3 with water.
3. Fill the grain insert with the pasta and water. Using the measuring bowl, fill the correlating heating tank to a level 3 with water.
4. Lock both bowls in place and turn babycook on.
5. Run steam cycle for both baskets.
6. Discard cooking juices and transfer the contents of the zucchini basket along with the basil and lemon juice into the blender and pulse in 3 second bursts until you reach your desired consistency.
7. Mix 1/2 of the vegetable puree with the cooked pasta and store the remaining puree for future use.
8. Sprinkle with parmesan and serve.

Instructions for Regular Cook Method

1. Chop the zucchini, asparagus and leek into 1" pieces. Roughly chop the basil.
2. In a medicum saucepan, bring 2" of water to a boil over medium heat. Place the zucchini, asparagus and leek into a steamer basket over the boiling water, cover, and cook for 15 minutes.
3. Meanwhile, cook pasta according to package directions.
4. Transfer the zucchini, asparagus and leek to a blender or food processor, add basil and lemon juice. Puree in short bursts until you reach your desired consistency.
5. Mix 1/2 of the vegetable puree with the cooked pasta and store the remaining puree for future use.
6. Sprinkle with parmesan and serve.

Notes

Yield: 12 ounces of chunky summer veggie pasta, 8 ounces extra chunky summer veggie sauce that can be stored in the fridge or freezer for future use.

Storage: 3 days in fridge, 3 months in freezer

Age: 6+ months for baby-led weaning or 9+ months for stage 3 baby food

Crispy White Fish with Pineapple & Avocado Chunks

An excellent way to serve fish to your toddler – seasoned to perfection and cooked until crispy on the outside yet still tender on the inside. Served with a side of pineapple and avocado chunks and cilantro brown rice for the win.

Course: Main Course | Cuisine: American

Prep Time: 5 Minutes | Cook Time: 12 Minutes

Servings: 4 Servings

Ingredients

For Fish

- 1 tbsp olive oil or butter
- 2 large filets of firm white fish cod, halibut, grouper or your favorite fish
- 1 tsp cumin
- 1/2 tsp ground cumin
- 1/4 tsp garlic powder
- 1/4 tsp mild chili powder

- 1/4 tsp pepper
- 1/2 lime

For Pineapple & Avocado Chunks

- 1/2 cup pineapple chopped
- 1 avocado peeled and cut into chunks

For Cilantro Rice

- 2 cups cooked brown rice warmed
- 1 tbsp butter or olive oil
- 1 tbsp fresh cilantro finely chopped

Instructions

1. Sprinkle both sides of the fish with the cumin, chili powder, garlic powder and pepper and rub into the fish with your fingers.
2. In a large skillet, heat olive oil over medium-high heat. Add in the fish and cook for about 4 minutes on the first side, or until brown. Carefully flip the filets and cook for roughly 2-3 minutes more, or until brown and crispy.

3. In a medium bowl, add in the pineapple chunks and avocado and gently toss.
4. In another medium bowl, take the warm cooked rice and add in the butter and cilantro. Stir until combined and butter is melted.
5. Serve the fish with a side of the rice and a small bowl of the pineapple and avocado chunks. Serve with a squeeze of lime.

Notes

Rice Options: you can use cooked brown, white or cauliflower rice in this recipe.

Yield: 2 small and 2 adult

Age: 9+ months

Family-Favorite Pumpkin Pasta

This easy and healthy Pumpkin Pasta can be made from scratch in only 15 minutes and with only 7 easy-to-find ingredients.

Course: Main Course | Cuisine: Italian

Prep Time: 2 Minutes | Cook Time: 13 Minutes

Servings: 8 Servings

Ingredients

- 16 ounce pasta, regular, gluten-free, lentil, chickpea, etc. (any shape you like)
- 1 tbsp olive oil
- 2 cloves garlic, minced
- 1 1/4 cup pumpkin puree
- 2 tbsp tomato paste
- 1 cup veggie or chicken broth
- 3-4 tbsp cream or canned coconut milk
- 1 tsp balsamic vinegar
- pinch nutmeg
- salt and pepper, to taste

Instructions

1. Bring a large pot filled with water to a boil and cook pasta according to instrucitons on package. Before straining, reserve 1 cup of pasta water.
2. Meanwhile, in a large saucepan pour in the olive oil and heat over medium heat. Add in the garlic and cook for 1-2 mintues, stirring often. Add in the pumpkin puree, tomato paste and broth and bring to a simmer, stir until combined. Reduce heat to low and add in the cream, balsamic vinegar, nutmeg and salt and pepper, stir and let simmer while pasta cooks.
3. Strain pasta and transfer to saucpan of pumpkin sauce. Stir in the pasta, adding the reserved water in 1/4 cup increments to thin out the sauce. I used the entire 1 cup of water for the recipe in the pictures above.
4. Spoon into bowls and sprinkle with parmesan (if using).

Notes

Age: great for baby-led weaning, toddlers, kids and adults – everyone will love this meal!

Storage: store leftover pasta in an air-tight container for 5 days in the fridge. Sauce can be stored for 5 days in fridge or 3 months in freezer. To defrost the sauce, simply leave in the fridge overnight or place frozen container of sauce in your sink filled with warm water, then heat on the stove.

To Make Vegan: use veggie broth and canned coconut milk. Skip the parmesan or use vegan parmesan.

To Make Gluten-Free: use any gluten free pasta you prefer. This is one of my favorite brands.

Cream or Coconut Milk: you can use either heavy whipping cream, half and half or canned full fat coconut milk in this recipe.

Kid-Friendly Pumpkin Risotto

This Kid-Friendly Pumpkin Risotto is a comforting dinner that the entire family will enjoy – from toddlers to grown-ups!

Course: Main Course | Cuisine: Italian

Prep Time: 3 Minutes | Cook Time: 30 Minutes

Servings: 8 Servings

Ingredients

- 4 cups chicken or vegetable stock or broth
- 1 cup canned pumpkin puree
- 2 tbsp unsalted butter or olive oil
- 1/2 white onion, finely diced
- 2 cloves garlic, minced
- 1 tsp dried thyme
- 1 1/2 cup Arborio rice
- 1/2 cup parmesan cheese, grated
- 1/4 tsp ground nutmeg
- black pepper

Instructions

1. In a medium saucepan, bring the stock and pumpkin puree to a boil over high heat, stirring until combined. Reduce to a simmer.
2. Meanwhile, in a large saucepan heat the butter or oil over medium heat. Add in the onion and garlic and let soften for 2-3 minutes. Add in the rice and thyme and cook for 2-3 more minutes or until the rice is just translucent on the outsides.
3. Add in 1-2 ladles of stock into the rice and stir. Let simmer until the liquid has evaporated, stirring occassionaly. Continue adding in ladles of stock, letting the rice simmer until the stock is evaporated and stirring until you have used up all of the stock and the risotto is creamy in texture – 20-25 minutes.
4. Add in the parmesan cheese and nutmeg and stir until combined. Season to taste with salt and pepper. I usually don't add any salt because the stock and parmesan are salty enough.
5. Serve immediatly and top with your favorite toppings.

Notes

Age: 9 months and up (use sodium-free or low-sodium for ages 9 months – 4 years). You can serve this to babies under 1 year as either a chunky puree or as a finger food that they can eat with a spoon or their fingers.

Yield: 6-8 servings

Storage: store in an air-tight container for up to 5 days in the fridge.

Fun Toppings

- goat cheese
- crispy sage
- candied or plain walnut or pecans
- parmesan cheese
- chopped bacon
- parsley
- rotisserie chicken
- pan-seared scallops
- cooked shrimp in lemon butter
- feta

Butternut Squash Mac N Cheese

Not only is butternut squash great for babies first puree, it makes a crave-worthy dinner for the entire family! You'll love this Vegan + Dairy Free Butternut Squash Mac and Cheese for toddlers and kids!

Servings: 8 Servings

Ingredients

- 1 medium butternut squash
- 12 ounces pasta, any shape
- 1 tbsp olive oil
- 1/2 yellow onion, diced
- 2 cloves garlic, minced
- 1 cup chicken or vegetable broth
- 1/2 tsp mild curry powder
- 1 tsp fresh thyme can also use sage or rosemary (optional)
- 1/2 cup grated parmesan cheese (optional)
- salt and pepper to taste

Instructions

1. Pre-heat oven to 400 degrees F. Line baking sheet with parchment paper or silicone mat.
2. Cut butternut squash in half, deseed and place on a baking sheet, skin side down. Bake for 40 minutes or until a fork can prick the skin easily.
3. Meanwhile, bring a large pot of water to a boil. Add pasta and cook according to the package directions.
4. In large skillet, heat oil over medium heat. Add onion and cook for 3-5 minutes. Add garlic and cook for an additional 2 minutes.
5. Scrape butternut squash from skin and place in blender or food processor. Add onion, garlic, thyme, curry and vegetable broth and puree until smooth.
6. Return pureed butternut squash to a skillet over medium heat. Add pasta, salt and pepper and stir until well combined.
7. Sprinkle with parmesan cheese, if desired, and serve immediately.

Notes

Age: great for 7+ months of age

Storage: in an airtight container in the fridge for up to 4 days

Healthy Chicken Nuggets with Green Bean "Fries"

Tender whole wheat chicken nuggets and crispy green bean "fries" are a perfect healthy alternative to the all-time favorite toddler meal.

Course: Main Course | Cuisine: American

Prep Time: 5 Minutes | Cook Time: 20 Minutes

Servings: 4 Servings

Ingredients

For Chicken Nuggets

- 1/2 pound chicken breasts, cut into bite-sized pieces
- 1/2 cup white whole wheat flour
- 1 tsp paprika
- 1 large egg
- 1/4 cup whole wheat Panko breadcrumbs
- 1/4 cup Parmesan, grated
- salt and pepper to taste (optional)

For Green Bean "Fries"

- 1/2 pound green beans, trimmed
- 1 tablespoon olive oil
- 1 tbsp parmesan cheese, grated
- 1 tbsp whole wheat panko breadcrumbs
- 1/2 tsp garlic powder

Instructions

1. Preheat the oven to 400 degrees F. Spray or line a baking sheet.
2. In a small bowl, mix together the flour and paprika. In another small bowl, whisk the egg. In another small bowl, mix together the breadcrumbs, parmesan cheese, salt and pepper (if using).
3. One at a time, add a piece of chicken to the flour and toss until coated, shaking off any excess flour. Then dip the chicken into the egg until coated. Then toss the chicken into the breadcrumb mixture until completely coated. Place the finished nugget on one side of the baking sheet. Continue this process

until all of the chicken pieces are coated and are on one side of the baking sheet.

4. In a medium bowl, toss together the green beans, oil, parmesan cheese, breadcrumbs and garlic powder. Place the green beans in a single layer on the other side of the baking sheet as the chicken nuggets.

5. Bake for 18-20 minutes, flipping half way through baking time, or until the chicken nuggets are golden brown and cooked all the way through.

Notes

Age: 1 year and up

Yield: makes 4 small servings

Freezer-Friendly: if freezing first, I would recommend prepping the chicken nuggets through step 3 and then placing them in the freezer in an air-tight baggie or container. When ready to eat, remove chicken nuggets from freezer, place on baking sheet and cook for 20 minutes.

Storage: in fridge for 5 days.

Gluten-Free: these can be made gluten-free by using a one-for-one gluten free flour (we love this brand) and gluten free breadcrumbs.

Spinach Waffles

This recipe for warm and wholesome waffles made with nutrient-packed spinach is perfect for baby 6 months and up.

Course: Baby Led Weaning | Cuisine: American

Prep Time: 10 Minutes | Cook Time: 15 Minutes

Total Time: 25 Minutes | Servings: 16 Small Waffles

Ingredients

- 2 cups white whole wheat flour (see notes below)
- 1 tbsp baking powder
- 1 tsp cinnamon
- 1/4 tsp salt
- 2 large eggs
- 1/2 cup milk
- 1/4 cup olive oil or melted coconut oil
- 1/4 cup applesauce or apple puree
- 1/2 tsp vanilla extract
- 1 cup packed spinach

Instructions

1. Preheat waffle iron to medium heat.
2. In a medium bowl, stir together the flour, baking powder, cinnamon and salt.
3. In a blender, add in the eggs, milk, oil, applesauce, vanilla extract and spinach. Blend for 1 minute on medium speed or until the spinach is completely blended.
4. Add the spinach mixture to the flour mixture and stir until just combined.
5. Pour waffle mixture onto waffle iron in 1/4 cup increments and bake according to waffle makers instructions.
6. Serve or store in an air-tight container in the fridge or freezer.

Notes

Age: 8 months and up

Freezer-Friendly: take any leftovers and place in a freezer zip-lock baggie and freeze. To reheat, place in toaster and toast until warm. The waffles will last 2-3 months in the freezer.

Notes on Flour: you can use all-purpose, white whole wheat or whole wheat flour in any combination that you prefer, I will usually use a combo of 1 cup all-purpose and 1 cup whole wheat or 2 cups white wheat flour. You can also make these gluten-free using a gluten-free flour mix. If using whole wheat flour, you may need to add in extra milk to thin it out as whole wheat flour is extra absorbent.

Printed in Great Britain
by Amazon